Published by Enna's Press
ISBN: 979-8-9945-835-9-3

Library of Congress Control Number: 2026905982

Art & Design: Created using licensed assets from Canva Pro.

For more books by the author, visit : iqralittlepages.com

JUVENILE NONFICTION / Concepts / Body
JUVENILE NONFICTION / Health & Daily Living / Diet & Nutrition

Printed in USA. First Edition 2026.

Note to Parents & Educators

Dear Grown-ups,

We all know that our bodies are amazing and we know that good food keeps them running. But how do we pass that knowledge onto our little ones in a way that actually sticks?

How do we make a carrot feel just as exciting as a cookie?

This book is your answer. It takes the wisdom you already carry and translates it into a world a child can understand and want to explore. From the mighty Brain down to the dancing Toes, we reveal the delicious foods that give each body part its power. We don't just teach children what to eat; we show them why their bodies deserve the best.

Our hope is that this book becomes a beloved favorite. A book they reach for at breakfast, lunch, and bedtime. A book that makes healthy choices feel less like a rule and more like a gift they give themselves.

Discover more books for amazing, confident kids at : iqralittlepages.com

Here's to growing strong, inside and out!

Sherifa E. Cudjoe
Author & Parent

For Yahya

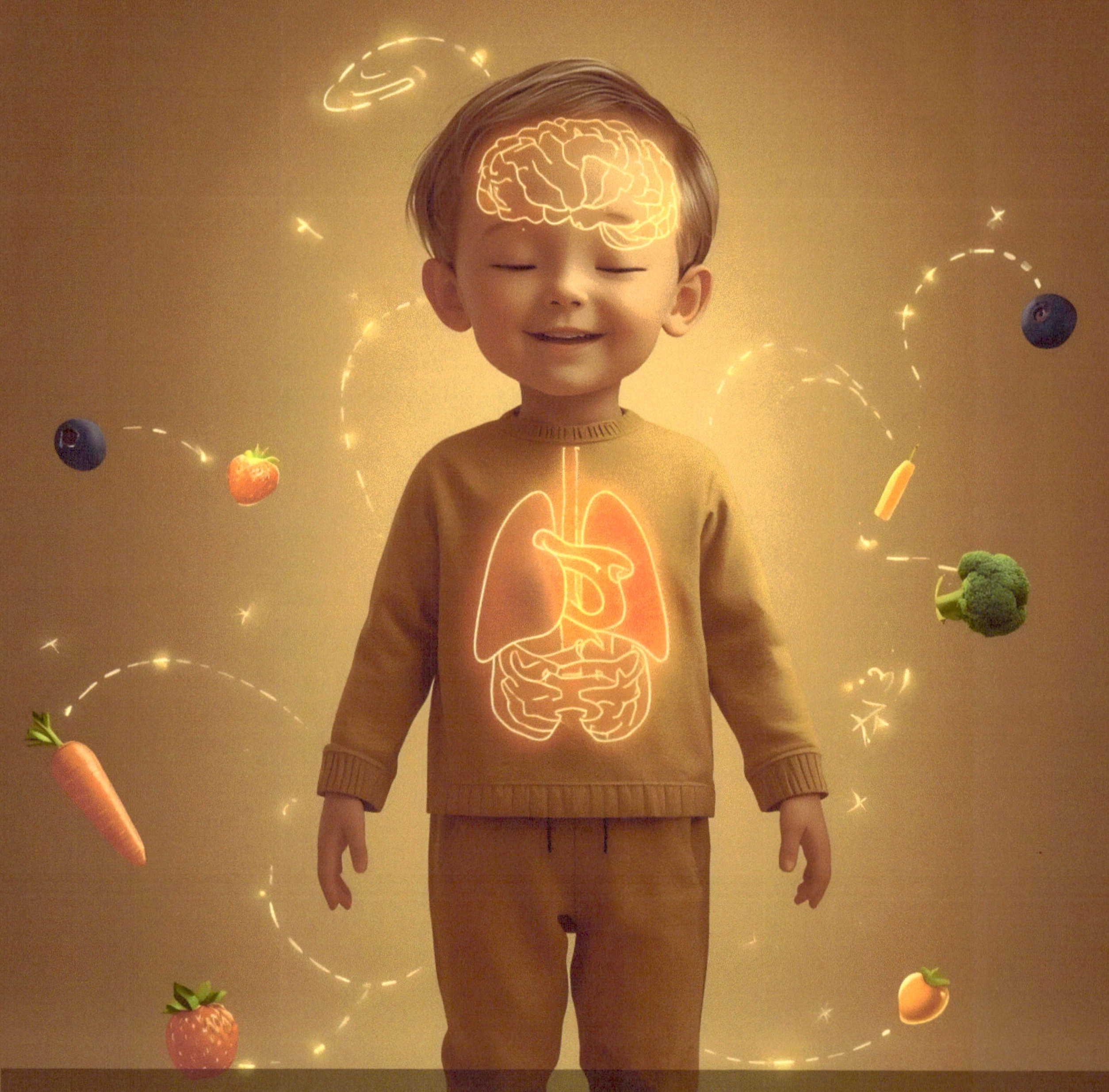

Look at you! Inside your body, amazing things are happening right now.

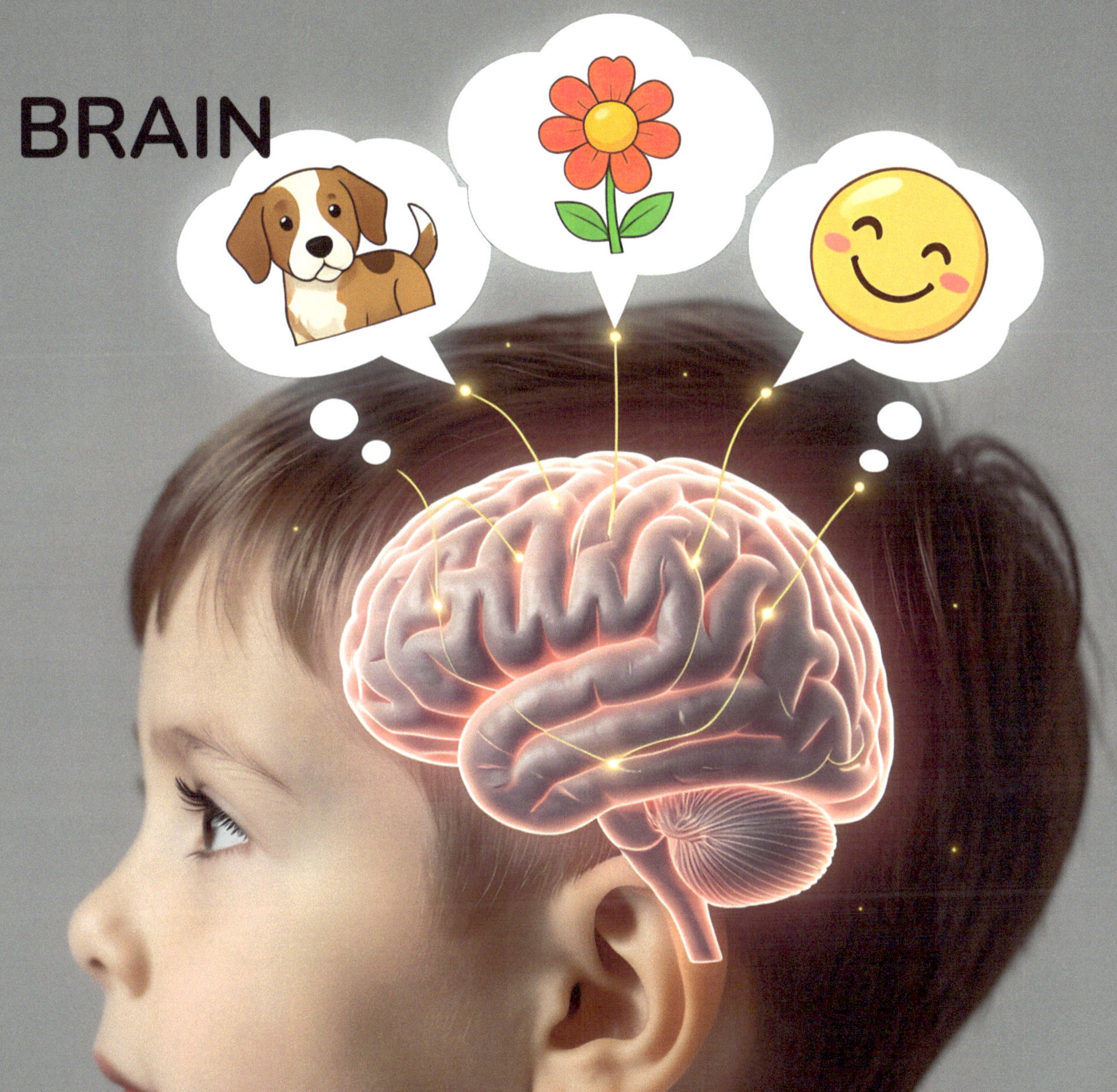

This is your brain. Your brain thinks your thoughts, keeps your memories, and tells your body what to do. Every time you learn something new, your brain grows stronger.

BRAIN

Blueberries
Eggs
Walnuts
Salmon
To keep your brain powerful: blueberries protect it.
Walnuts help you think. Salmon helps it grow.
Eggs help you remember.

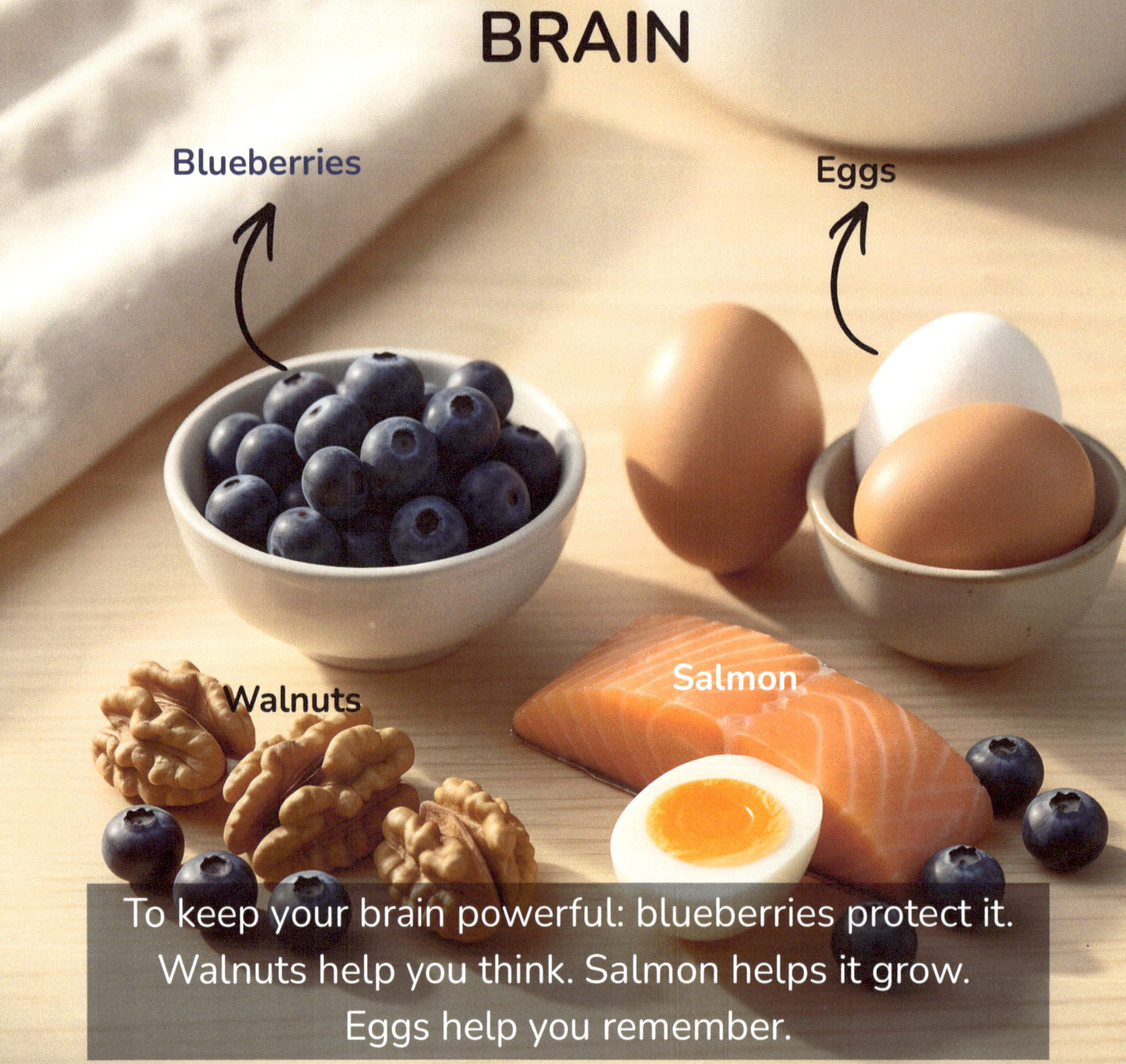

EYES

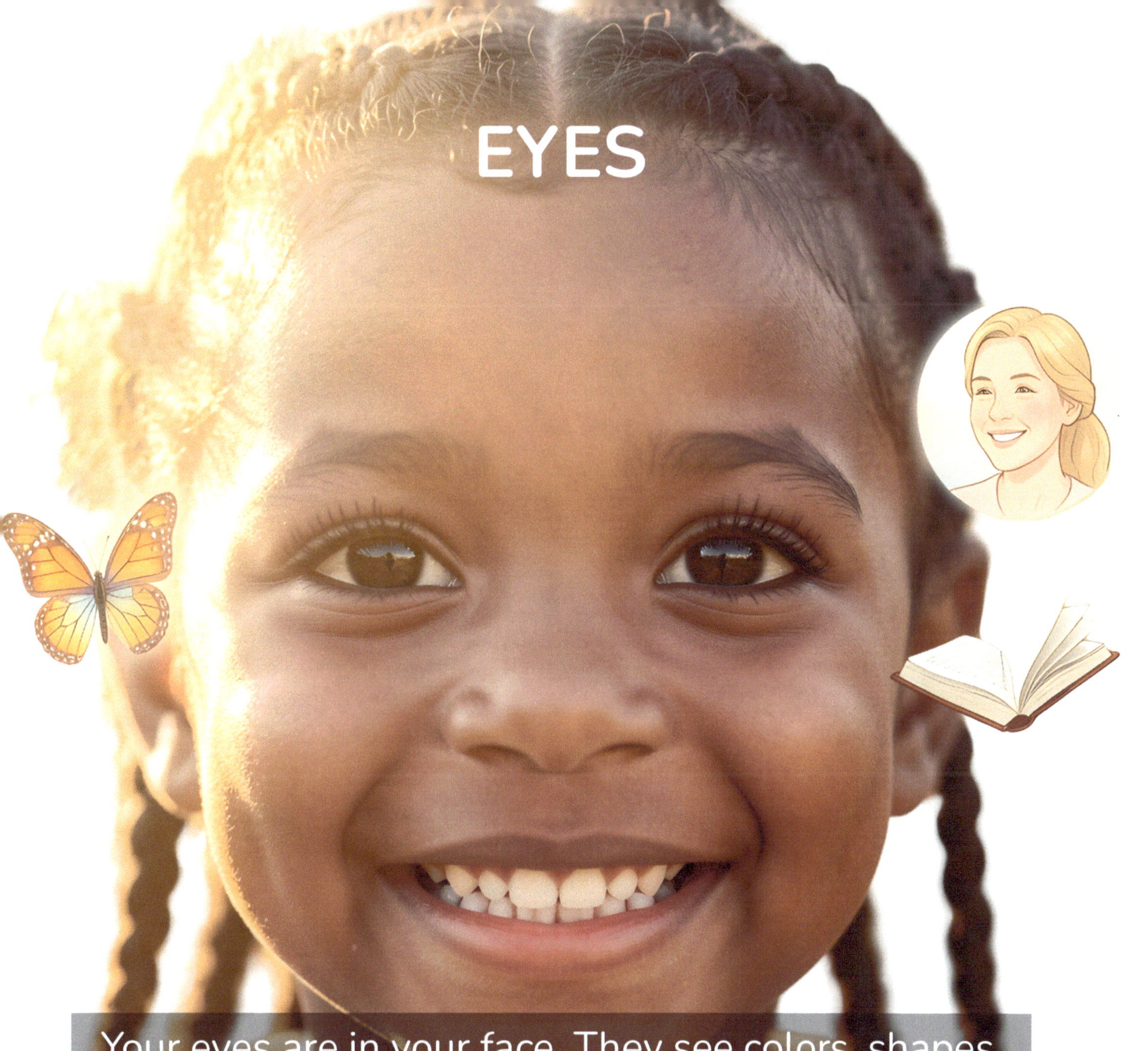

Your eyes are in your face. They see colors, shapes, faces, and light. They help you explore the world.

EYES

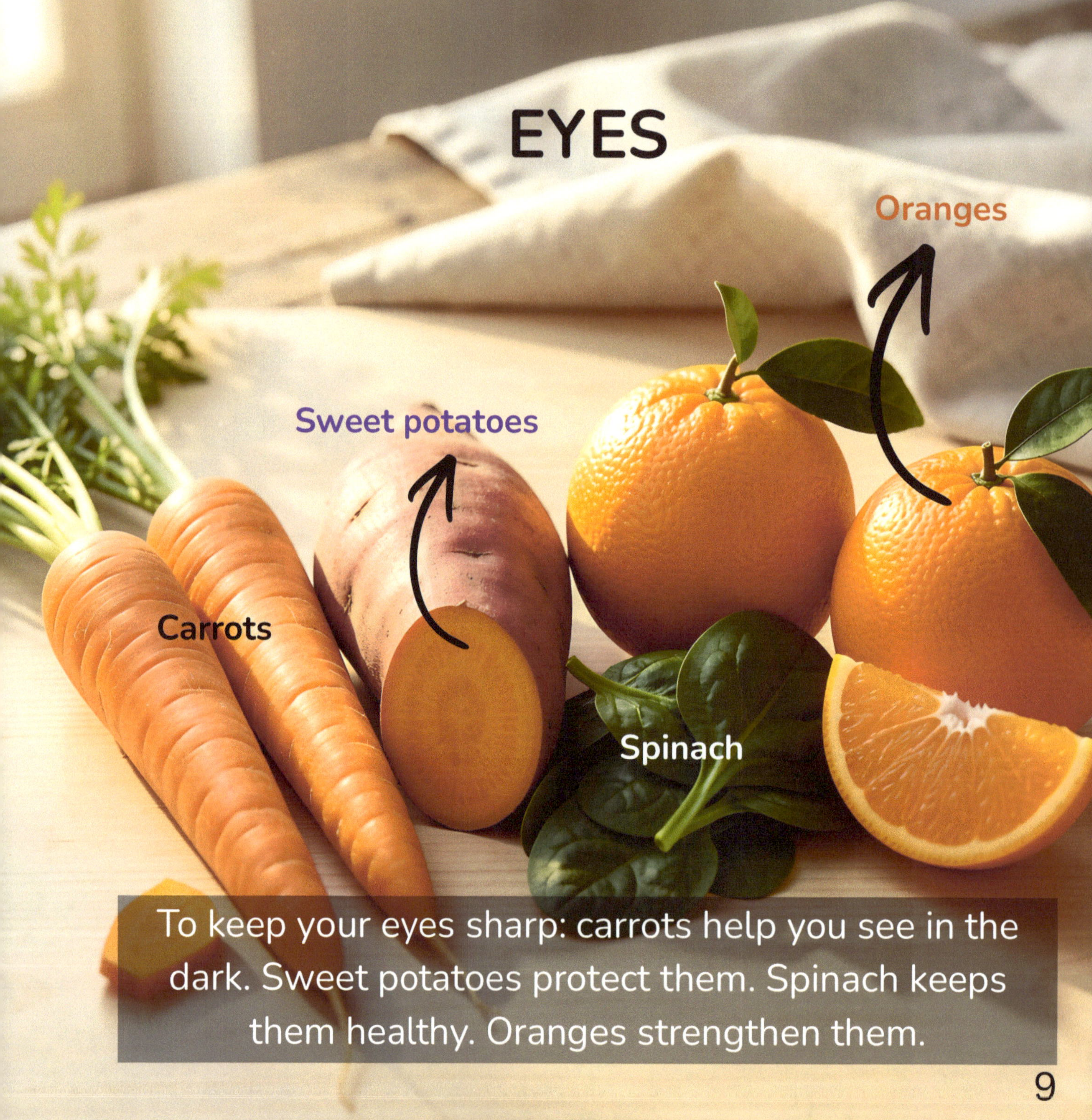

To keep your eyes sharp: carrots help you see in the dark. Sweet potatoes protect them. Spinach keeps them healthy. Oranges strengthen them.

EARS

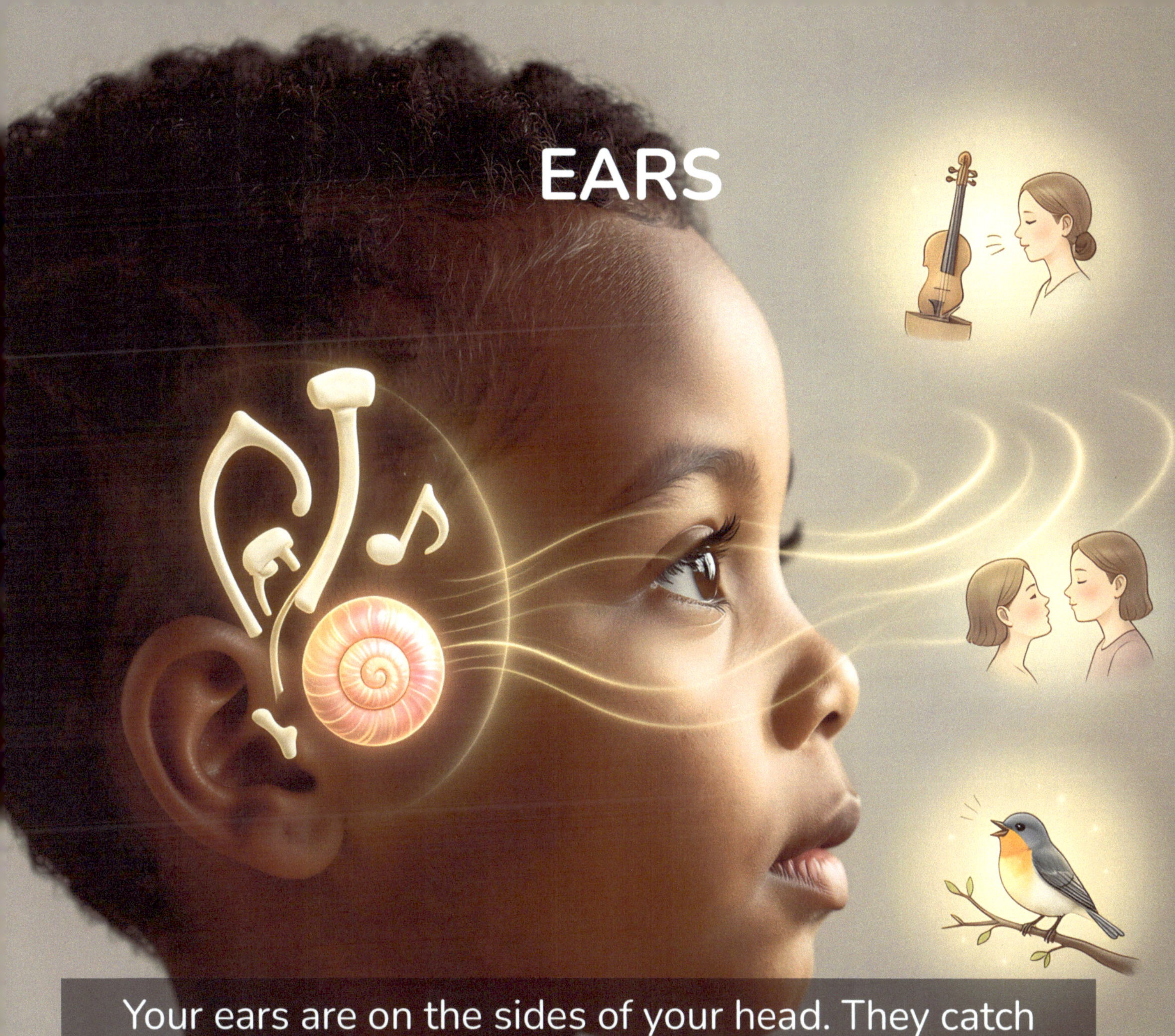

Your ears are on the sides of your head. They catch sounds; loud and soft and send messages to your brain.

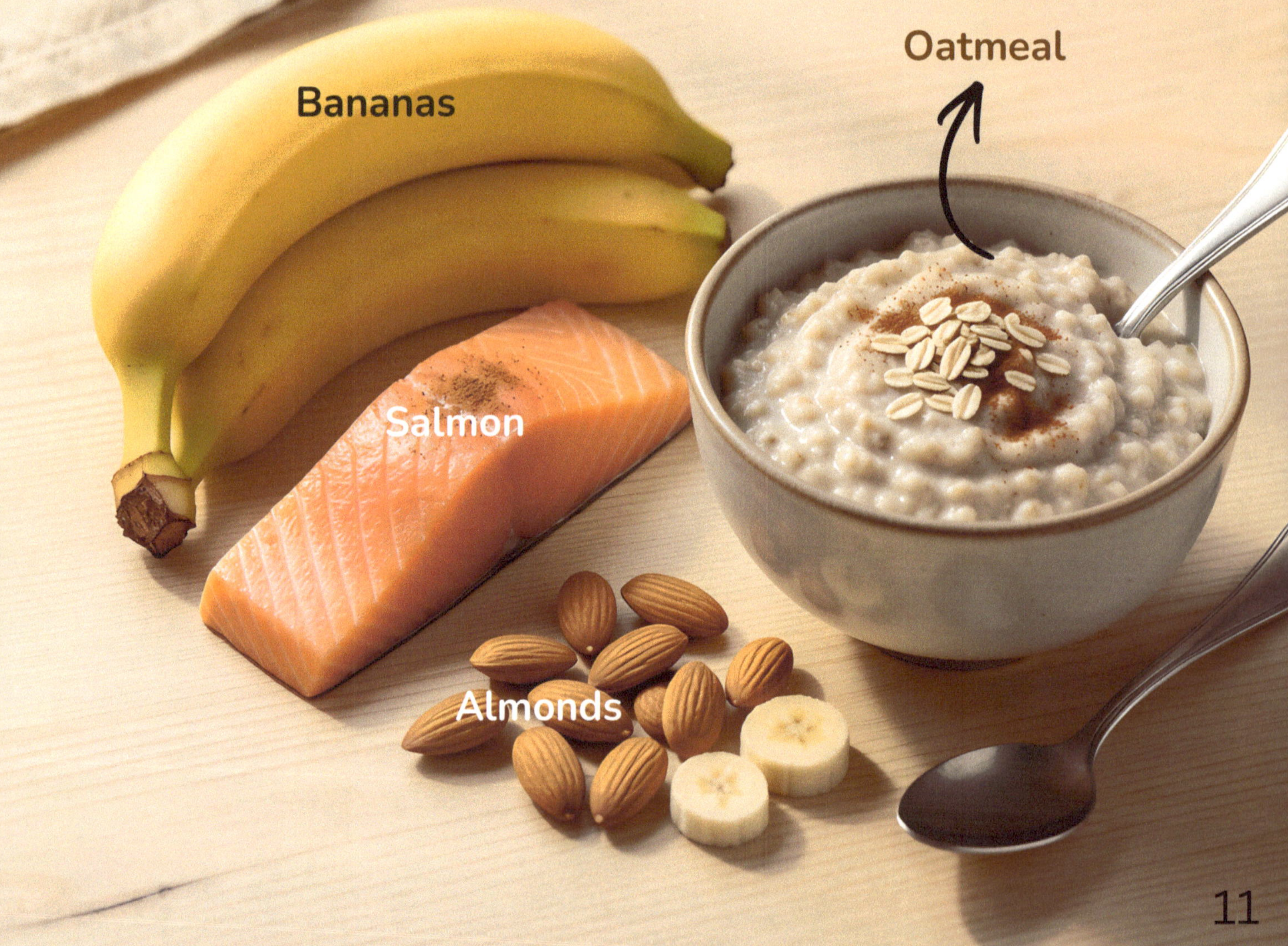

To keep your ears hearing well: bananas protect hearing nerves. Salmon keeps the inner ear healthy. Almonds help blood flow. Oatmeal gives steady energy.
Bananas
Oatmeal
Salmon
Almonds

NOSE

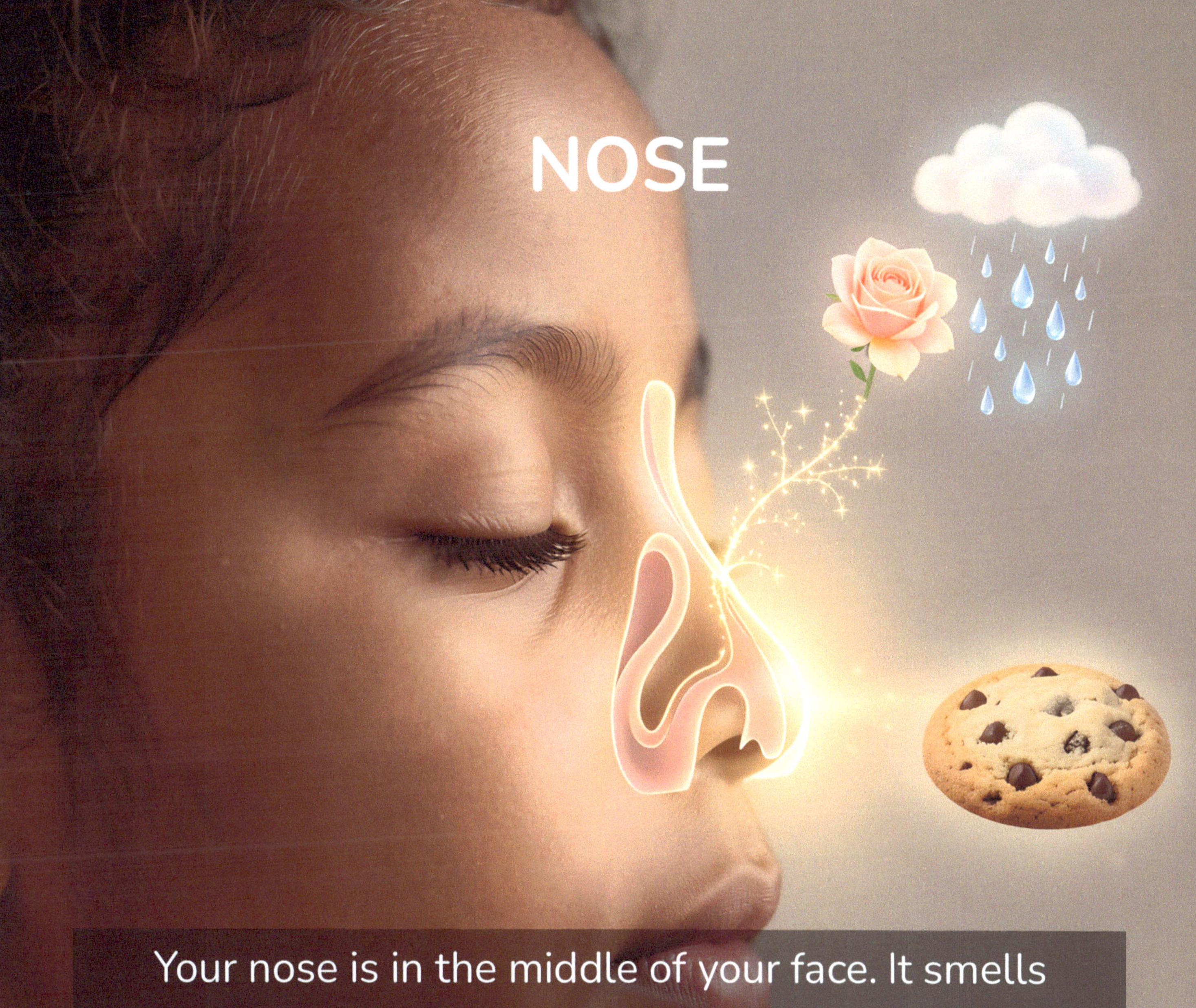

Your nose is in the middle of your face. It smells flowers, food, and fresh air. It also warms and cleans the air you breathe.

NOSE

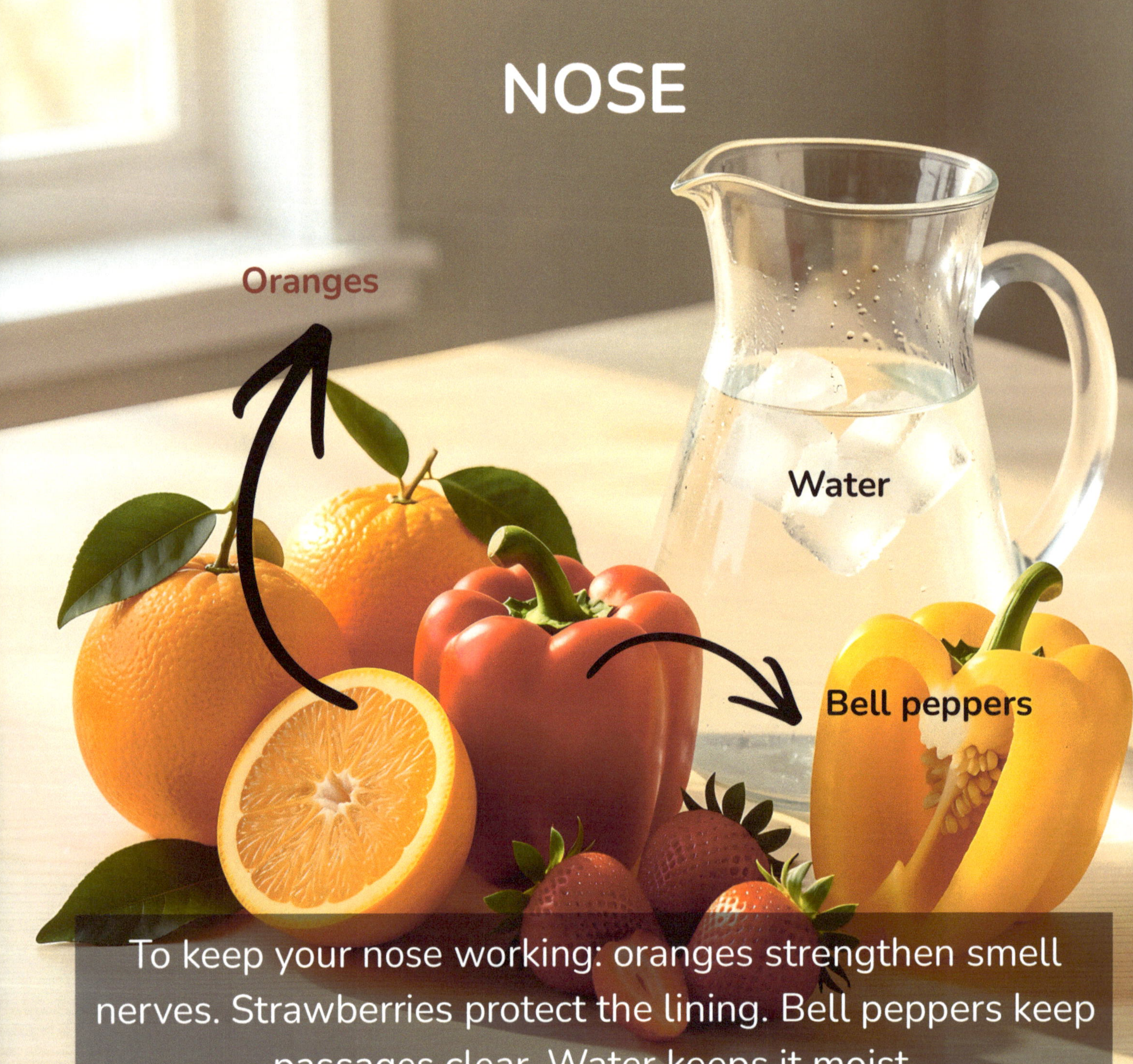

To keep your nose working: oranges strengthen smell nerves. Strawberries protect the lining. Bell peppers keep passages clear. Water keeps it moist.

TEETH

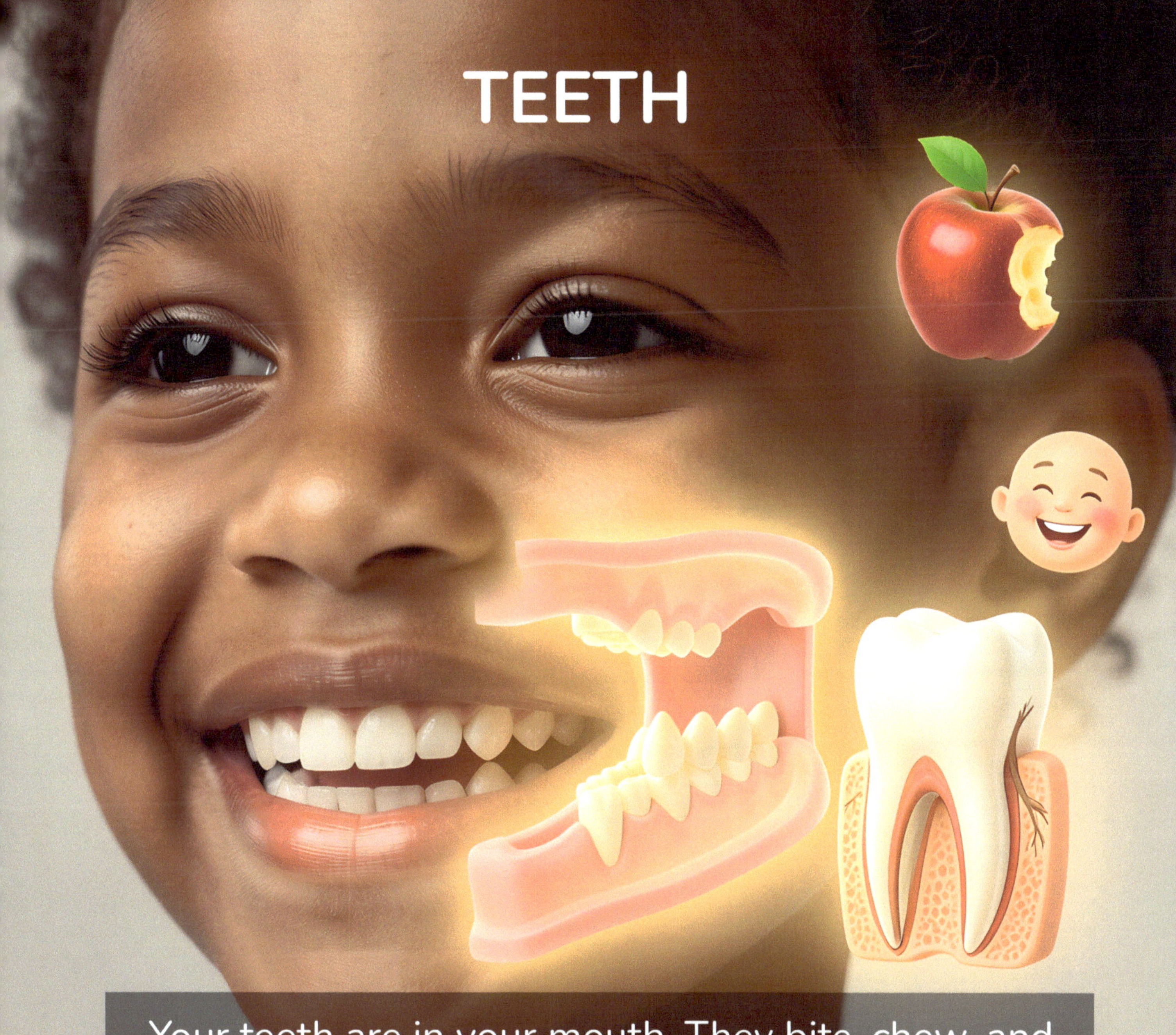

Your teeth are in your mouth. They bite, chew, and help you speak. Strong roots hold them in place.

TEETH

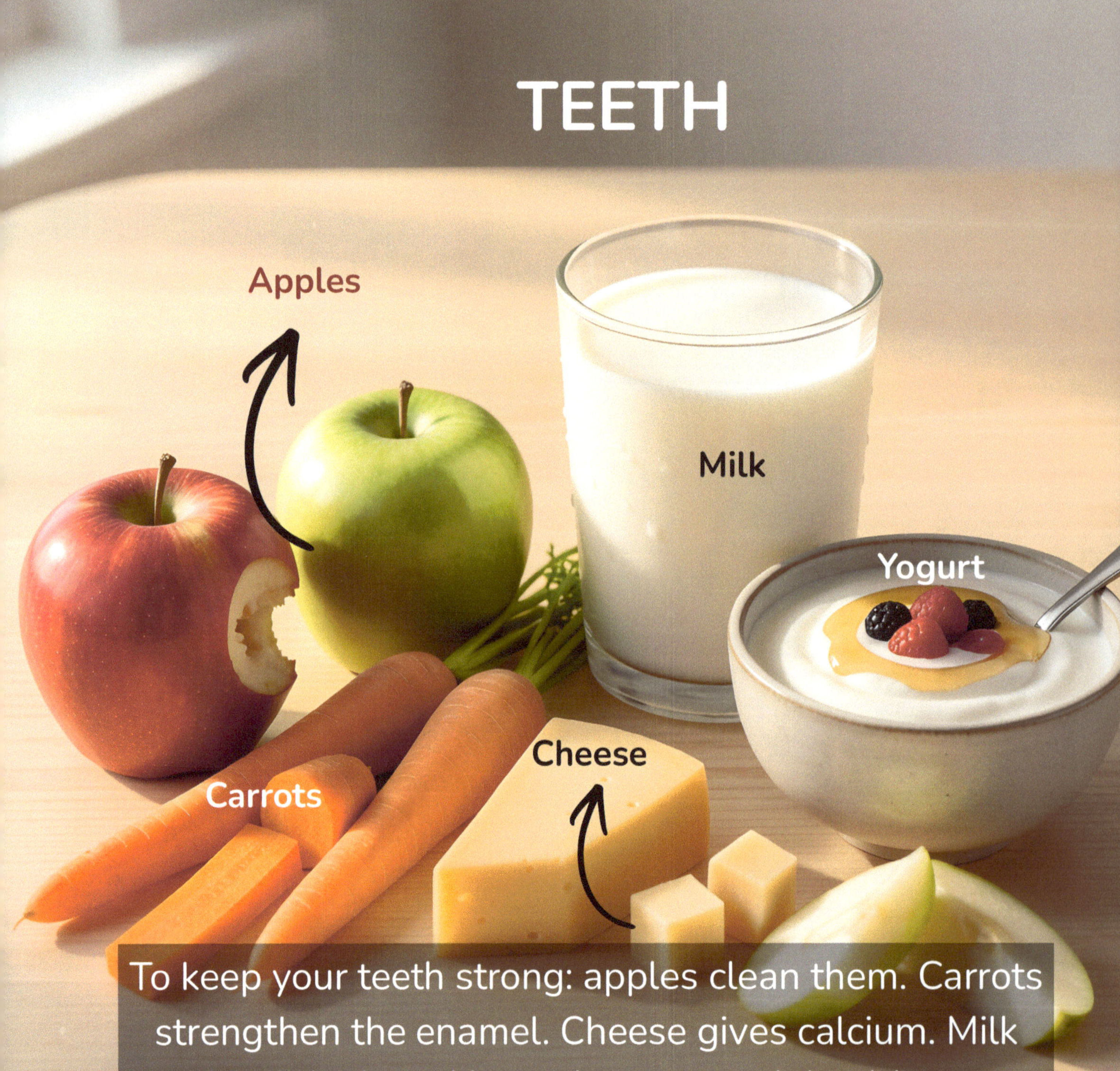
Apples
Milk
Yogurt
Cheese
Carrots
To keep your teeth strong: apples clean them. Carrots strengthen the enamel. Cheese gives calcium. Milk builds them. Yogurt keeps mouth healthy.

HEART

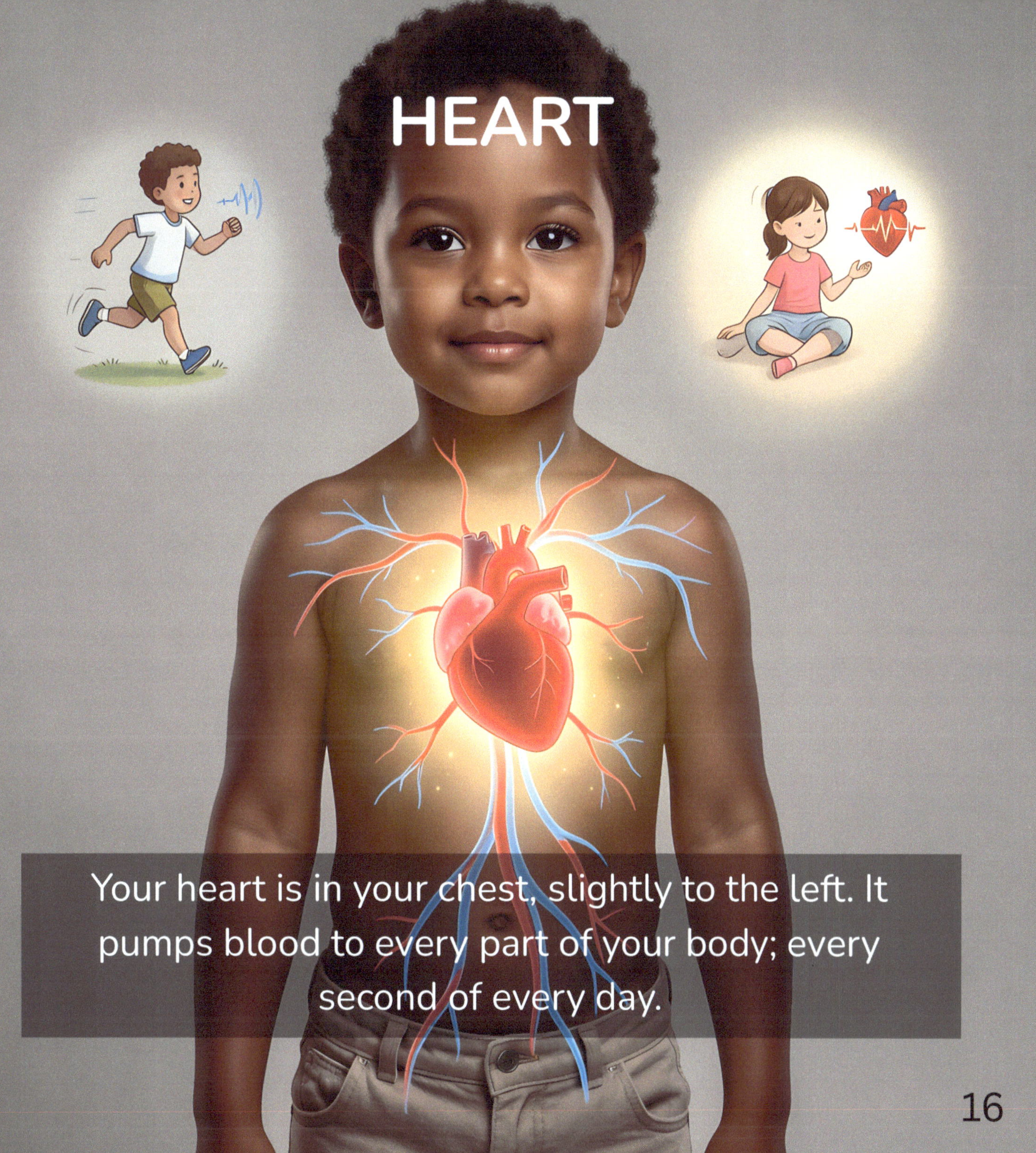

Your heart is in your chest, slightly to the left. It pumps blood to every part of your body; every second of every day.

16

HEART

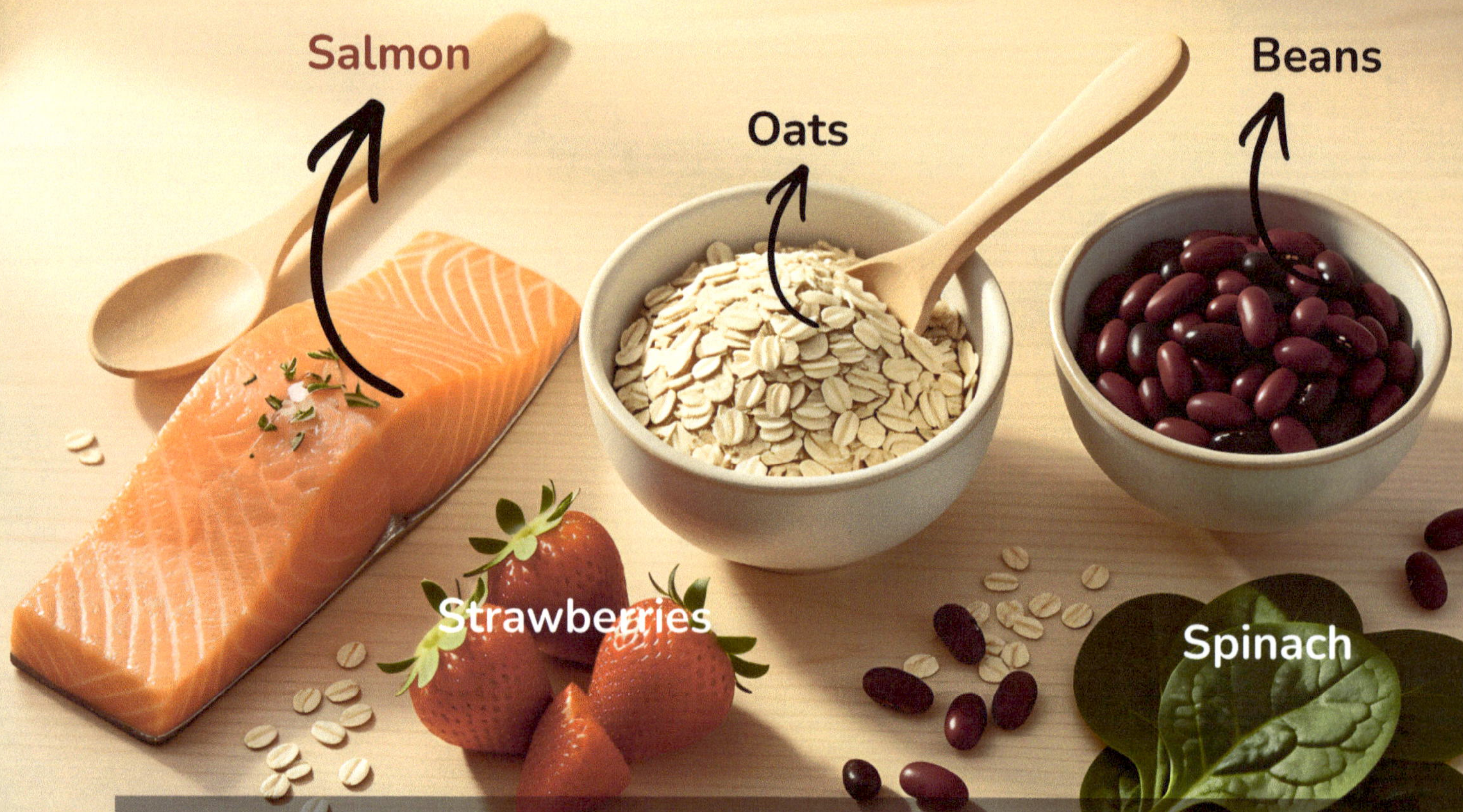

To keep your heart pumping strong: salmon gives healthy fats. Strawberries protect it. Oats clean blood vessels. Beans give steady energy. Spinach helps heart muscles.

LUNGS

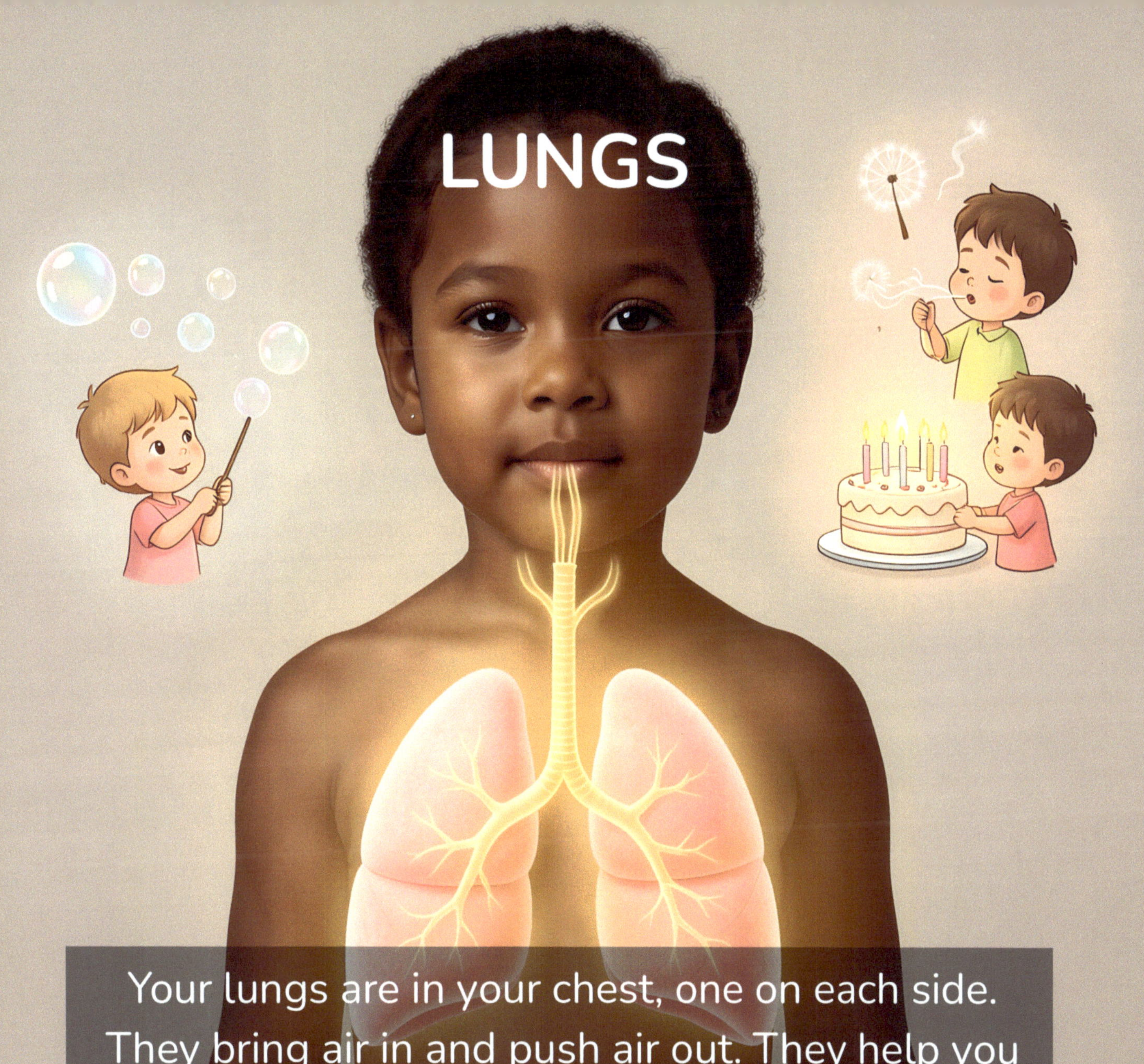

Your lungs are in your chest, one on each side. They bring air in and push air out. They help you breathe, blow, and shout.

LUNGS

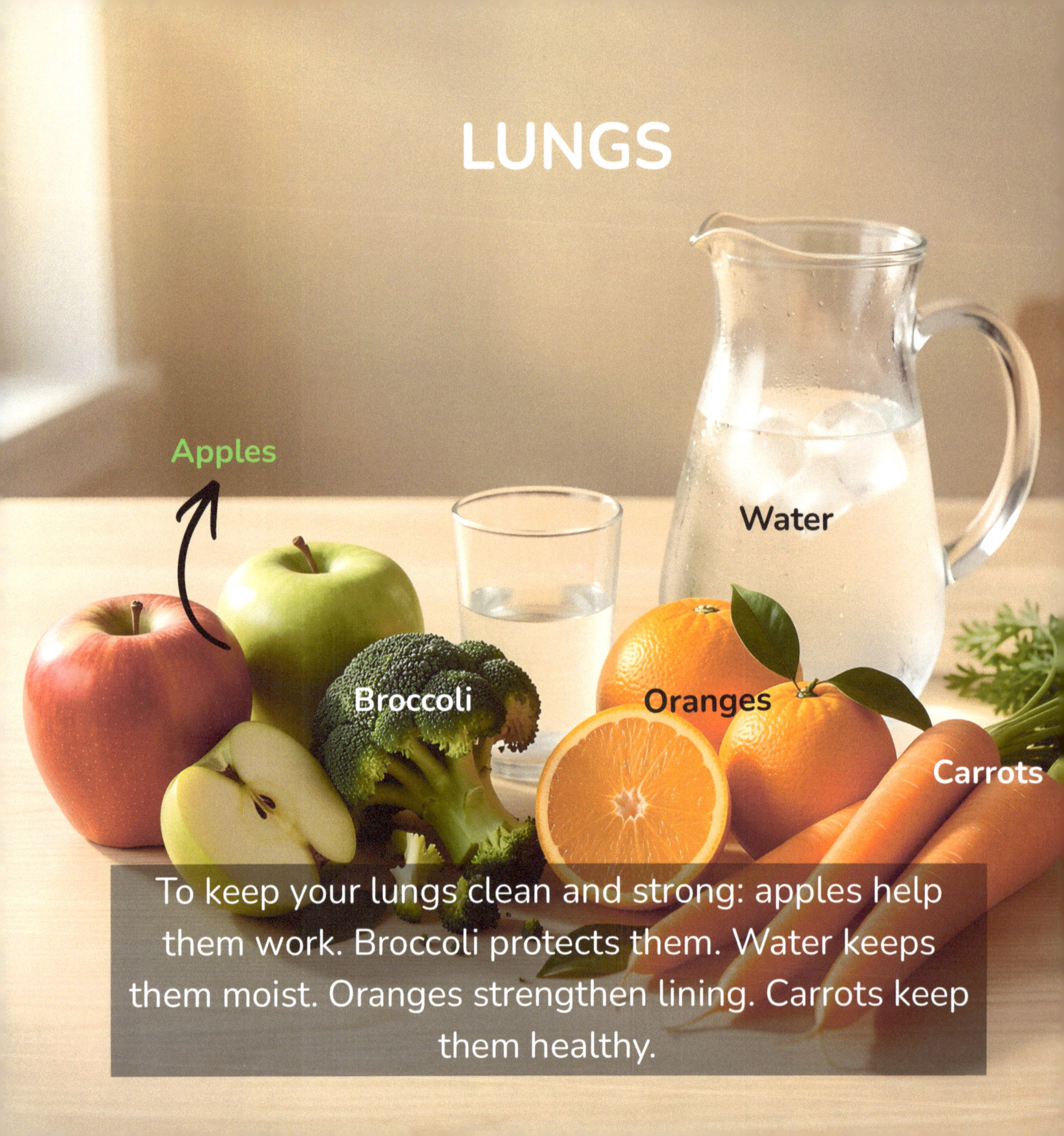

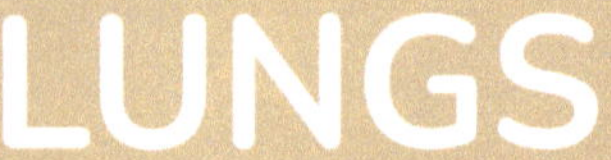

To keep your lungs clean and strong: apples help them work. Broccoli protects them. Water keeps them moist. Oranges strengthen lining. Carrots keep them healthy.

STOMACH & INTESTINES

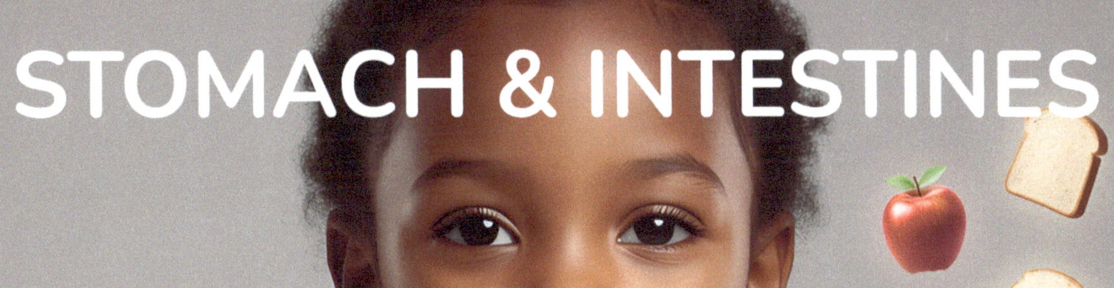

Your stomach and intestines live in your belly. Food goes in, gets mixed up, and your body takes what it needs for energy.

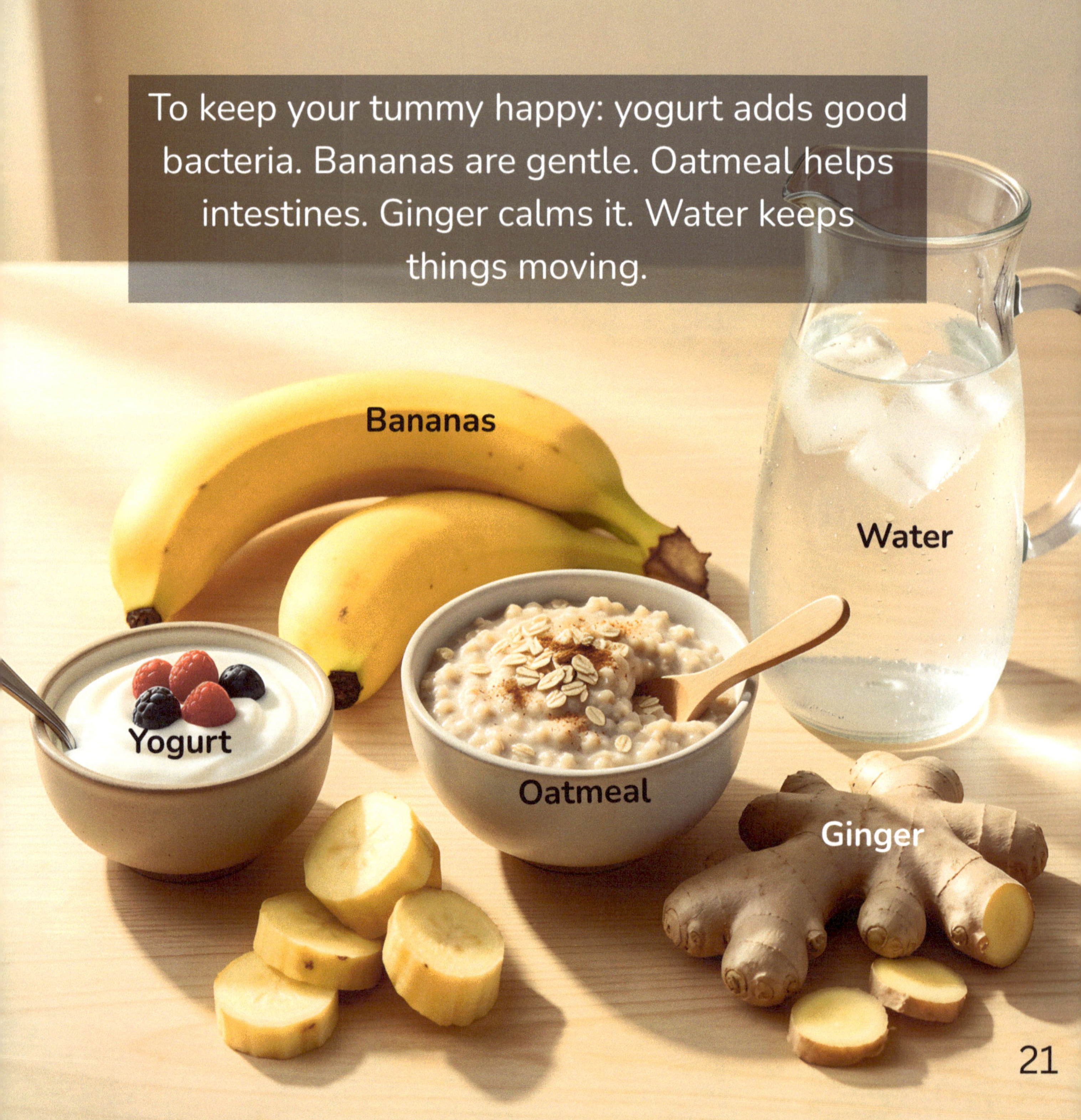

To keep your tummy happy: yogurt adds good bacteria. Bananas are gentle. Oatmeal helps intestines. Ginger calms it. Water keeps things moving.
Bananas
Water
Yogurt
Oatmeal
Ginger

BONES

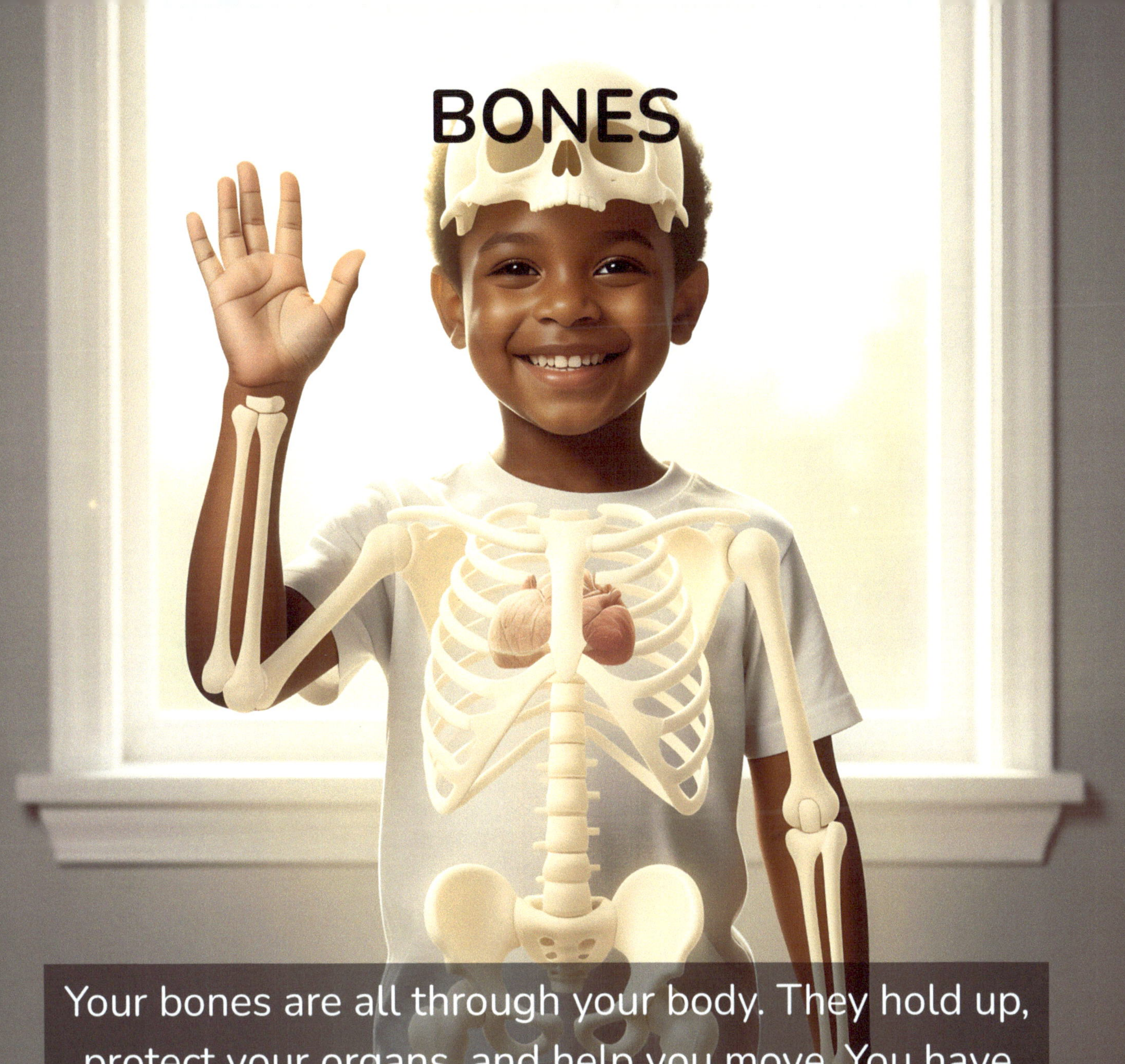

Your bones are all through your body. They hold up, protect your organs, and help you move. You have over 200 bones!

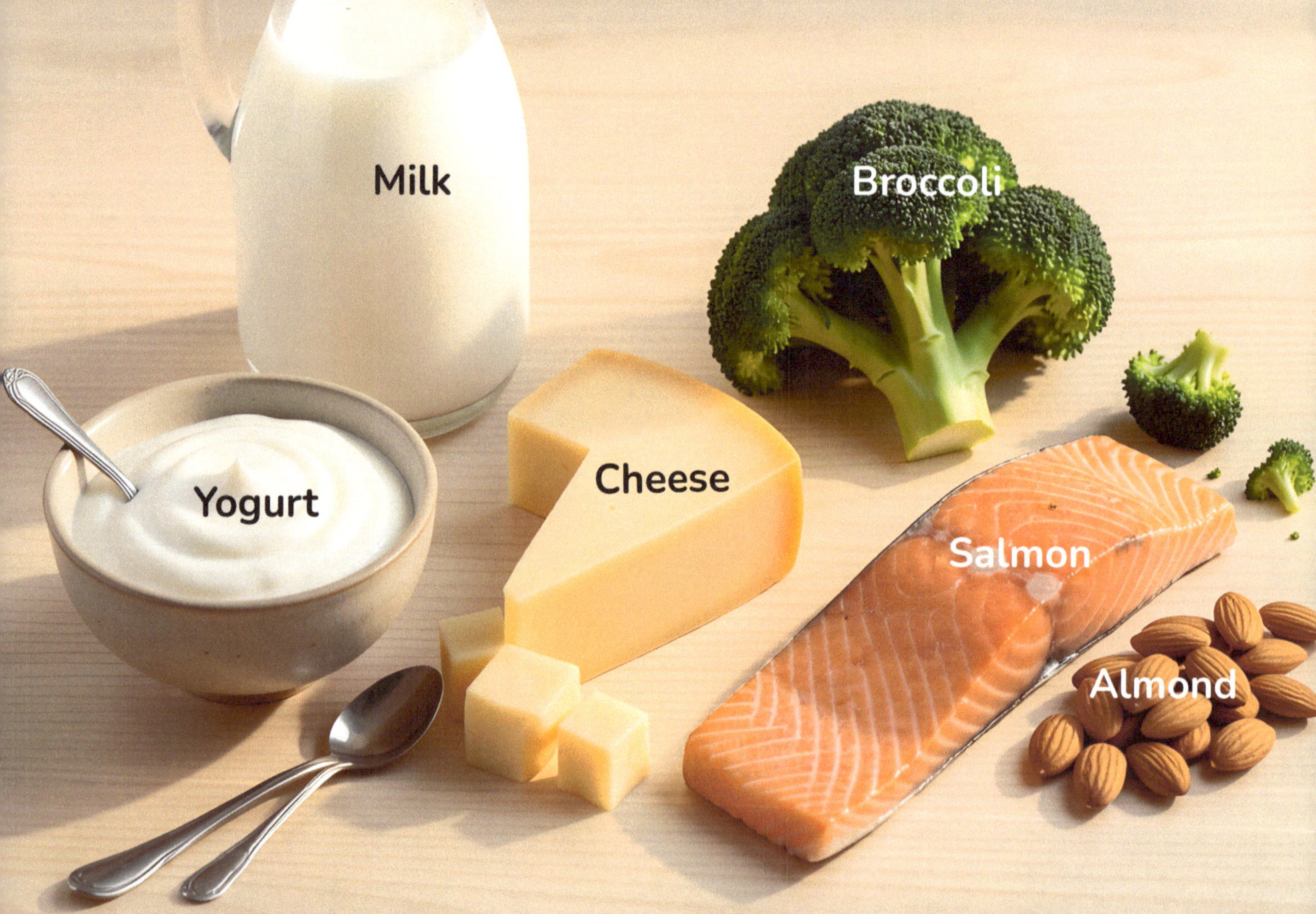

To keep your bones strong: milk builds them. Yogurt keeps them hard. Cheese strengthens them. Broccoli gives vitamins. Salmon helps absorb calcium. Almonds add minerals.
Milk
Broccoli
Yogurt
Cheese
Salmon
Almond

MUSCLES

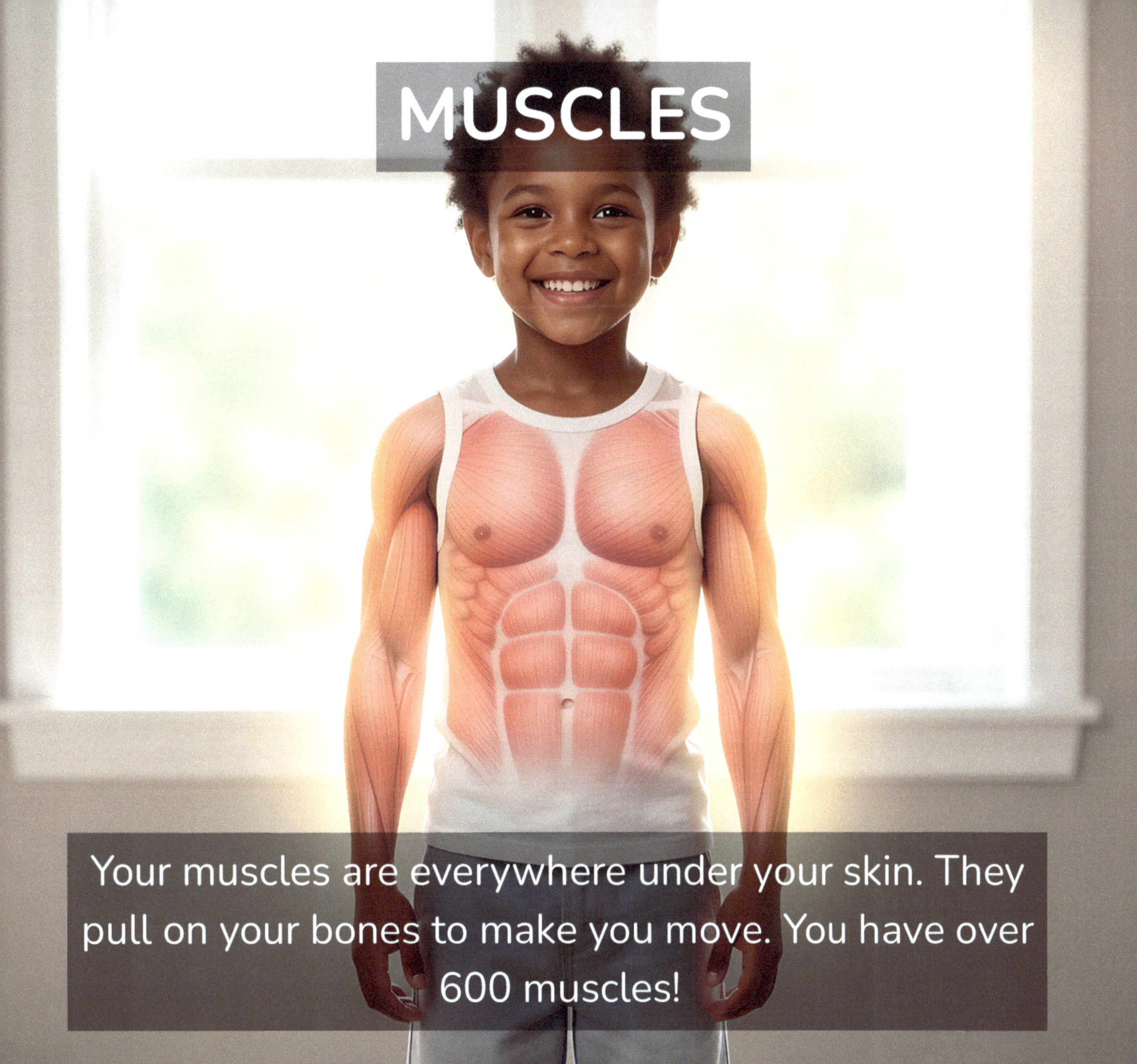

Your muscles are everywhere under your skin. They pull on your bones to make you move. You have over 600 muscles!

MUSCLES

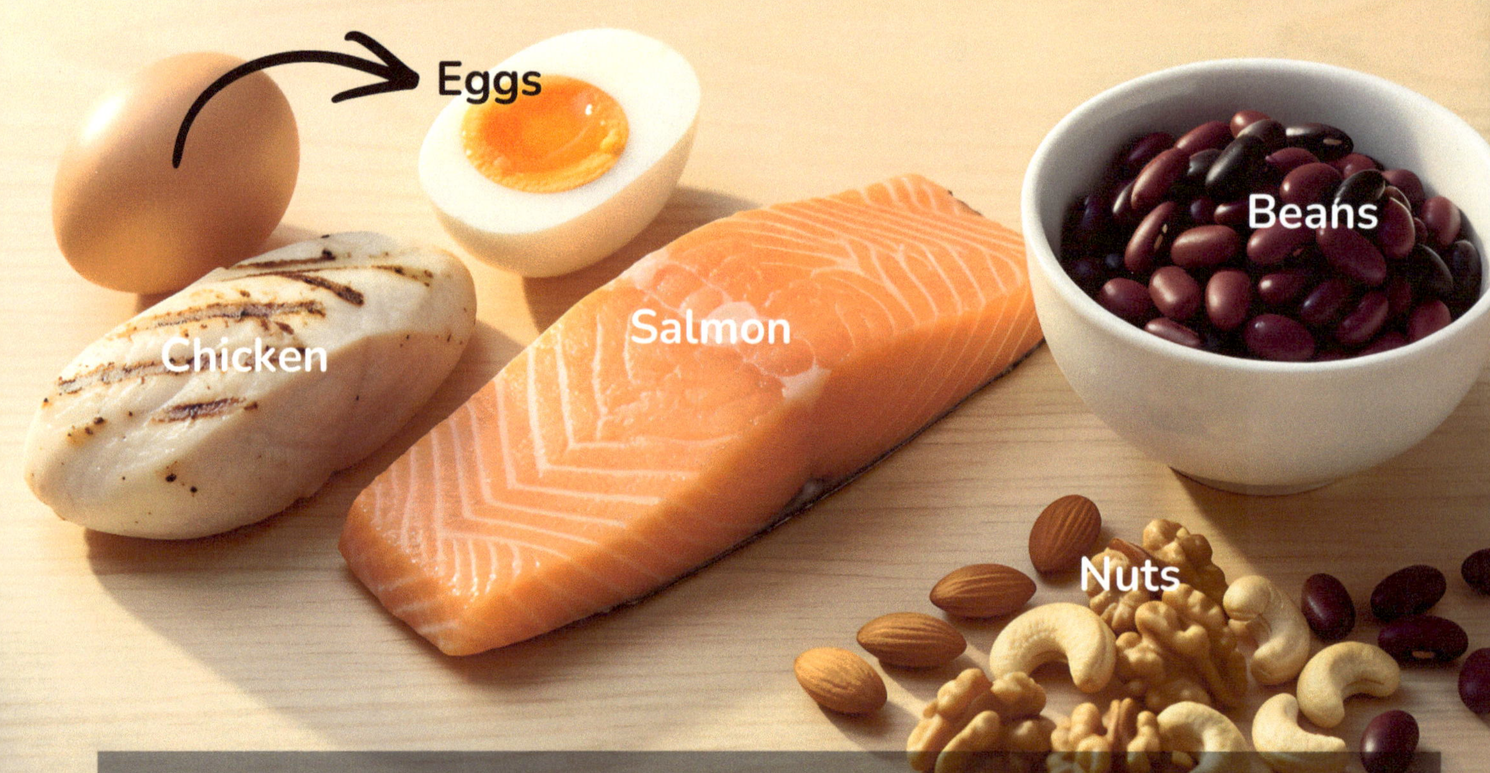

To keep your muscles strong: chicken builds them. Eggs repair them. Fish fuels them. Beans give energy. Nuts add protein.

SKIN

Your skin covers your whole body. It protects everything inside. It feels warm, cool, soft, and ticklish.

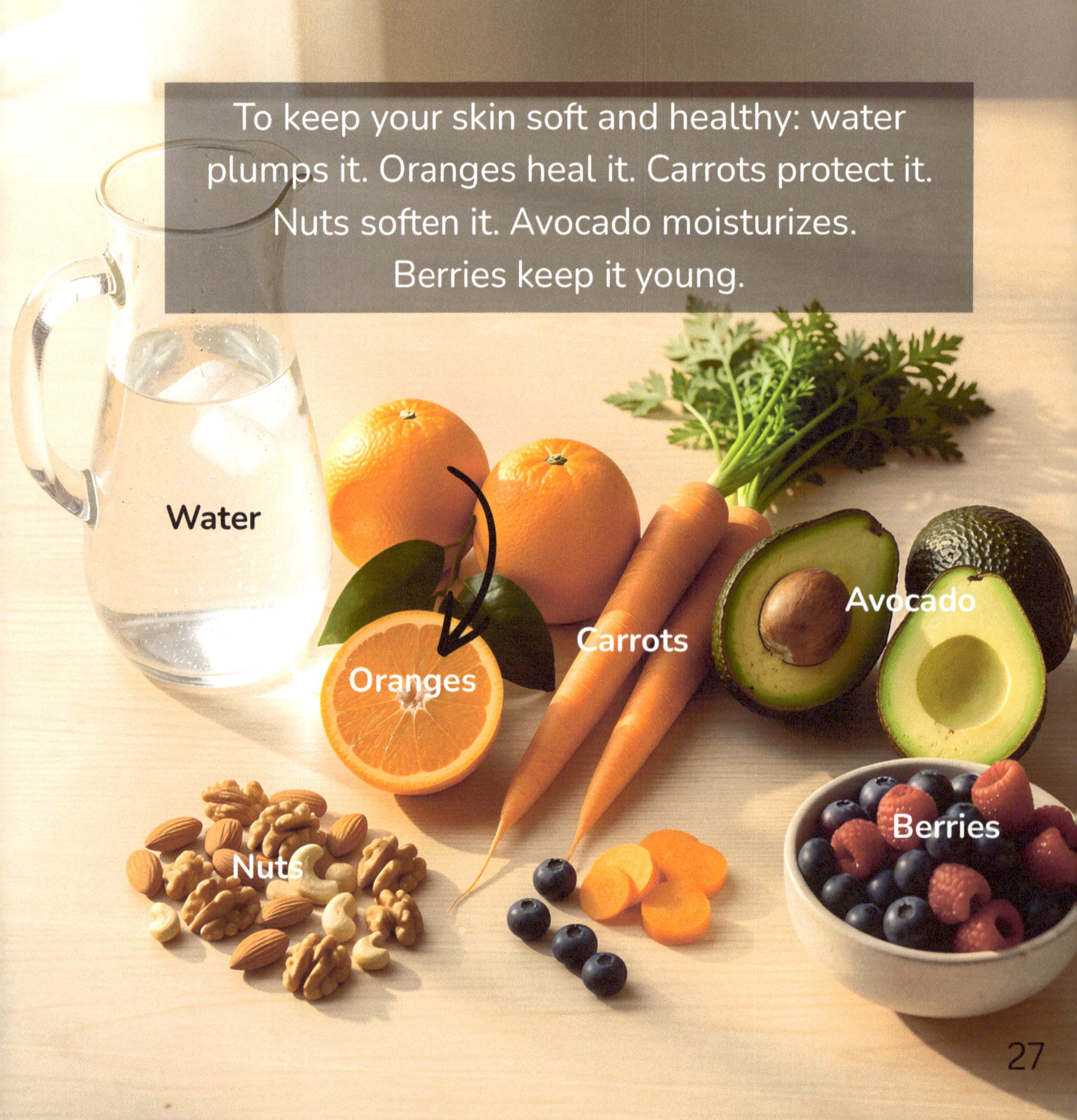

To keep your skin soft and healthy: water plumps it. Oranges heal it. Carrots protect it. Nuts soften it. Avocado moisturizes. Berries keep it young.
Water
Oranges
Carrots
Avocado
Nuts
Berries

TOES (AND FEET)

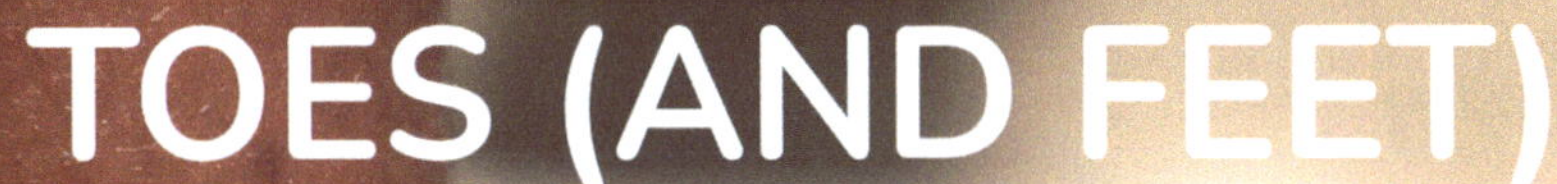

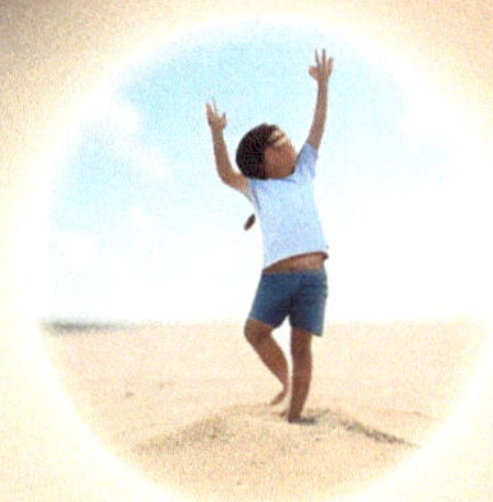

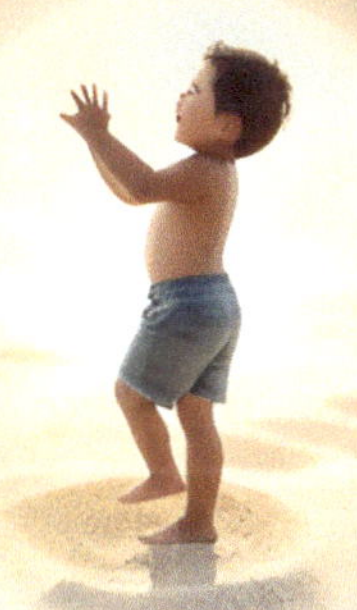

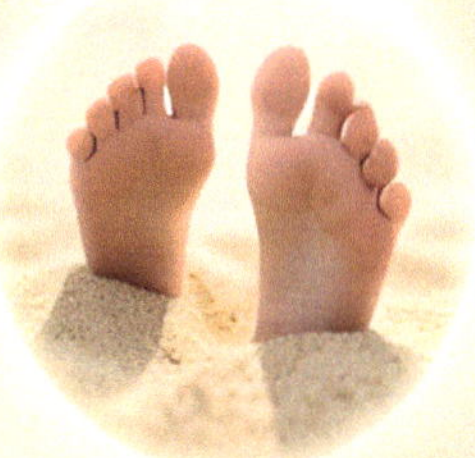

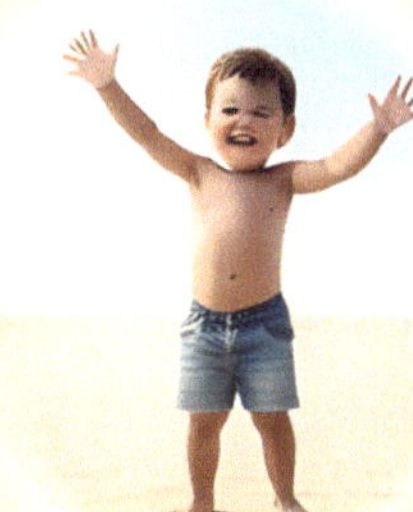

Your toes are at the ends of your feet. They help you balance, walk, run, and wiggle. Tiny bones let them move.

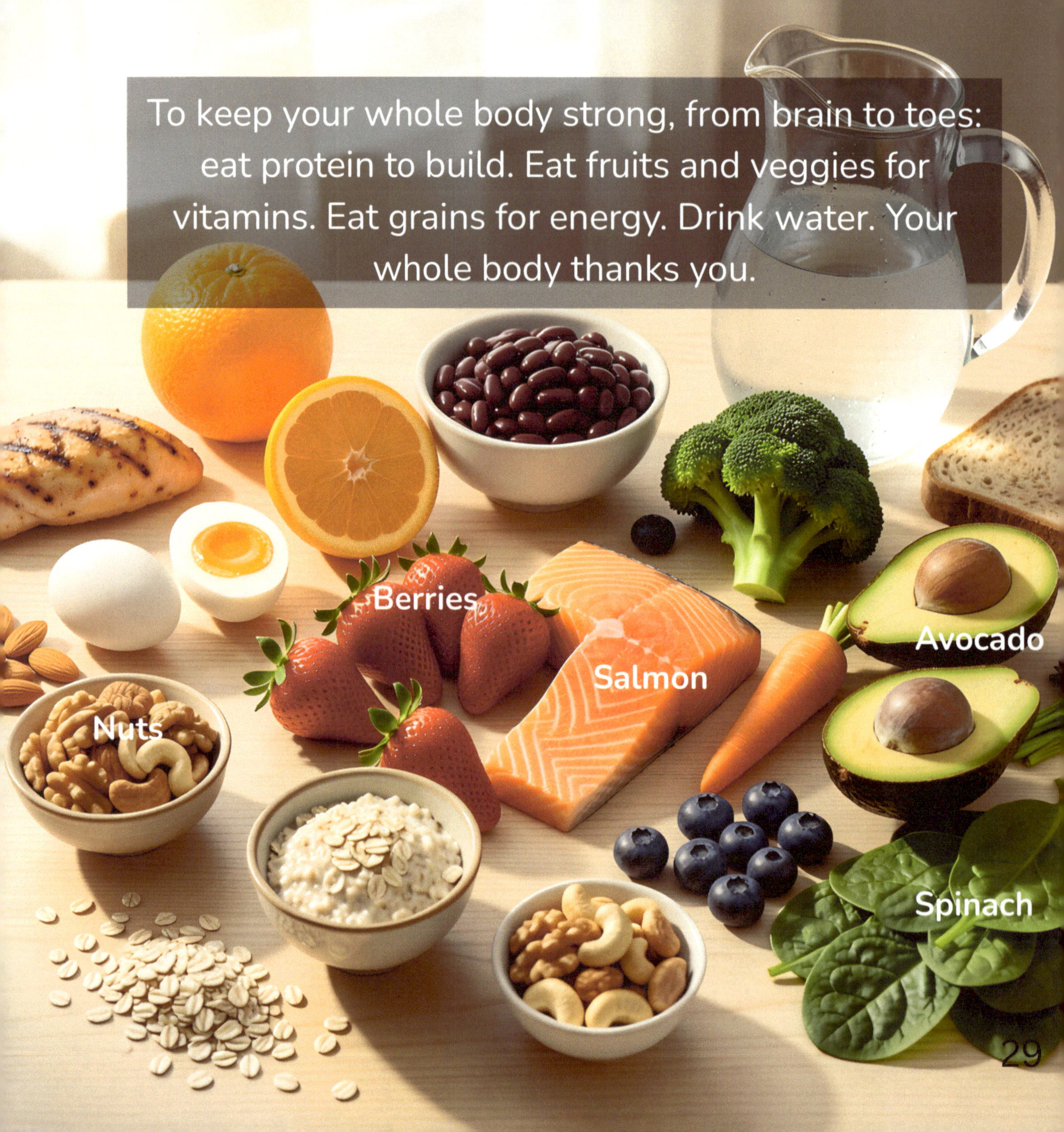

To keep your whole body strong, from brain to toes: eat protein to build. Eat fruits and veggies for vitamins. Eat grains for energy. Drink water. Your whole body thanks you.
Berries
Nuts
Salmon
Avocado
Spinach
29

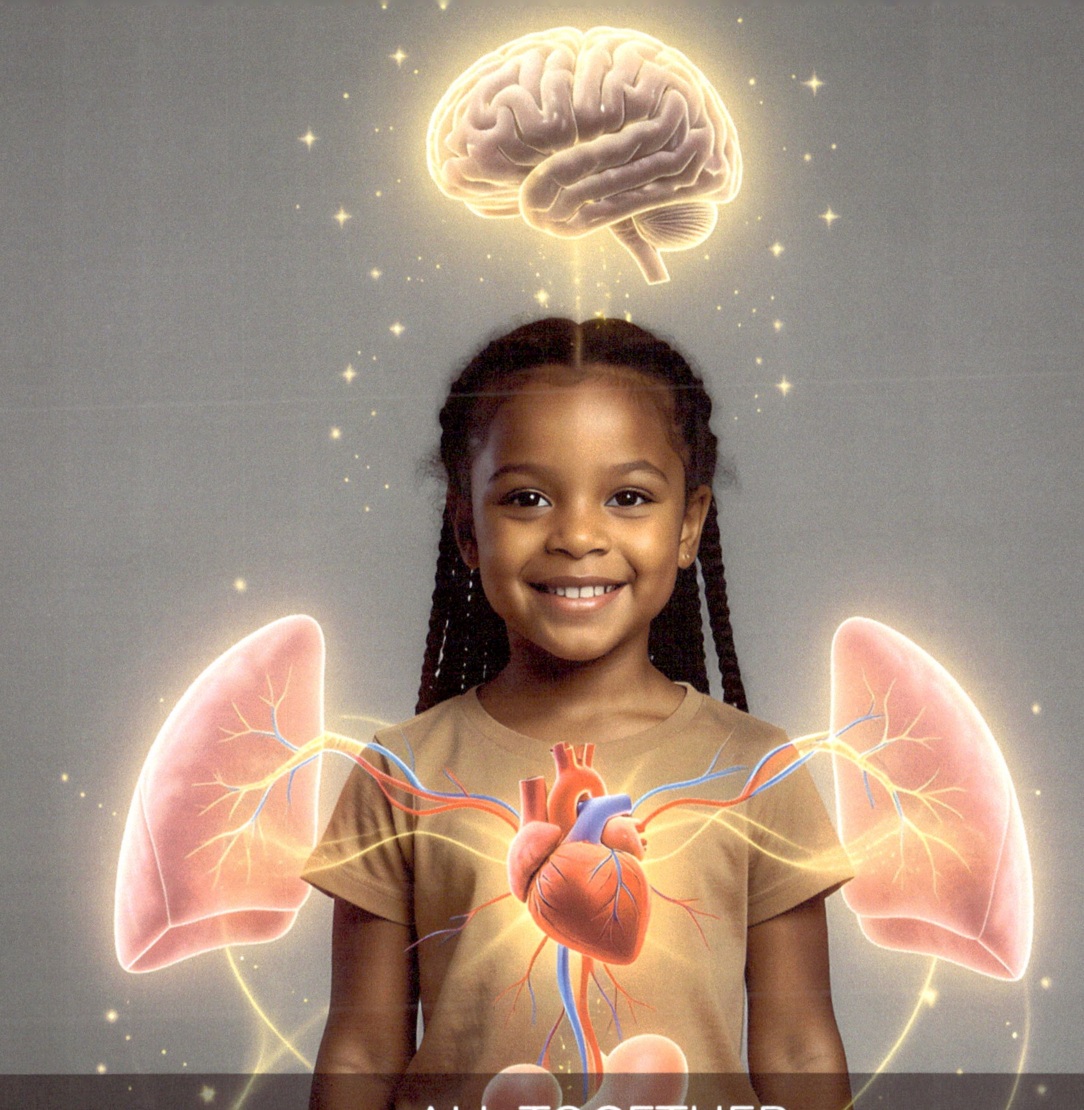

ALL TOGETHER:
Look at you. Every part works together. Your brain
thinks. Your heart pumps. Your muscles move.
Your bones hold. Your skin protects. Your toes
wiggle. You are amazing.

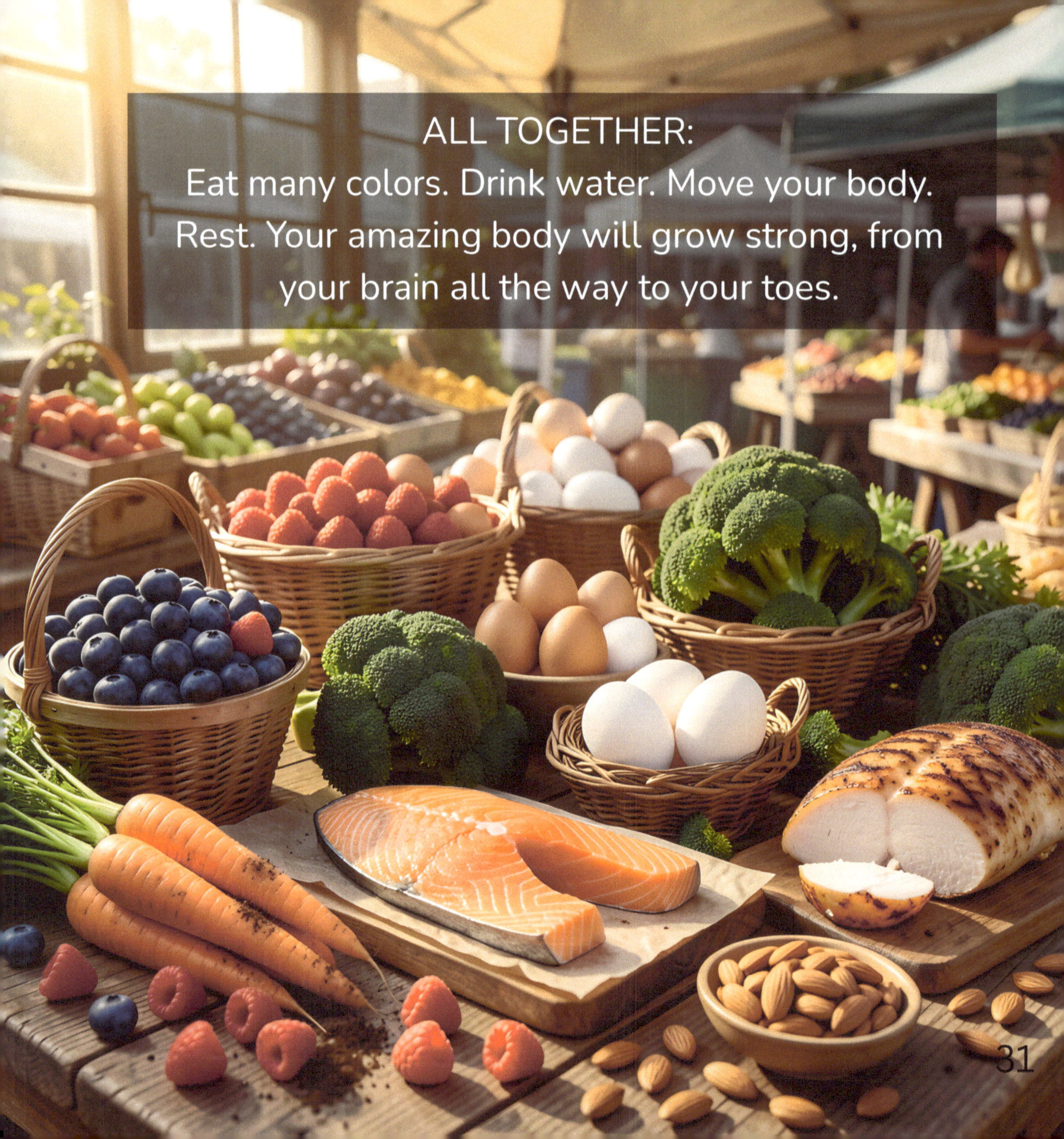
ALL TOGETHER:
Eat many colors. Drink water. Move your body.
Rest. Your amazing body will grow strong, from
your brain all the way to your toes.